The

D.O.P.E.

Director of Pharmacy Education for the
Hospital Pharmacist

Authored by Todd R. White, Pharm.D., R.Ph.

Index

Introduction

In an ideal world a pharmacist filling the position of Director of Pharmacy (DoP) in a hospital setting would come well versed in Hospital Pharmacy finance, operations, law, accreditation, clinical skills, management skills, communications skills and be an overall well rounded leader. The reality is that there are not a plethora of perfect candidates to be out-of-the box perfect DoPs. Often times the DoP is a well meaning staff pharmacist who steps up to the challenge of being the Director when senior management asks them to fill the spot as an Interim Director; only to find out there is no such position as Interim Director. Others may be recruited from a non-hospital based pharmacy practice without hospital pharmacy experience or appropriate training to be the new DoP. Unfortunately the DoPs that are given the title by default, or accept the position without experience and/or sufficient training often struggle and fail. The duties of a DoP are so diverse that without the proper training and mentoring the pharmacist becomes overwhelmed and discouraged, which leads to resignation or self-demotion.

It takes a certain personality type to be successful at directing a Hospital Pharmacy. They have to be open-minded to new ideas and suggestions from other. Their work ethic has to be second to none. Directors have to work with other Departmental Directors, Senior Executives, and physicians who may have very strong personalities. This requires excellent verbal and written communication skills to be able to affect change.

This book was written to assist new DoPs in learning their day-to-day duties and to give some insight in to dealing with hard situations and difficult people. Some of the ideas are skills that need to be developed to manage people as well as processes, and others are helpful hints to manage the workload of a DoP. Understanding the role of a DoP early on and not having to learn on the job, will improve the new DoP's chance to succeed in this challenging career choice.

Chapter One

Finance

Dealing with financial issues is a daily duty of the DoP. Performing these daily duties requires a working understanding of accounting processes, terms, regulations and workflows. Financial processes are set by the Chief Financial Officer (CFO) and managed by the Controller. The Controller is the Lead Accountant whose role is to control all accounting day-to-day activities.

The Controller oversees the Pharmacy Department's revenue and expenses. Payroll also falls under the Controller's stewardship, which will affect the DoP's productivity and human resource responsibilities. Duties of the Controller may be delegated to a staff Accountant, so the DoP needs to know the chain of communication.

It is important to know who the CFO and Controller are of the organization and what their roles are as they relate to pharmacy operations. The DoP should have an organizational chart available and know the organization's hierarchy.

The CFO is a senior management position in charge of all aspects of financial regulation and operations. CFO's report to the Chief Executive Officer (CEO) and oversees Accounting and Business operations departments, including supply chain management and purchasing contract compliance. Although the Pharmacy Department is not routinely directly managed by the CFO, he/she does require the DoP to report daily financial activity reports, monthly budget compliance and productivity reports, as well as annual inventory reports. Budget development, both capital and operational, is responsibilities of the CFO. The DoP will meet with the CFO annually to discuss departmental budgetary needs for capital equipment and operation expenses. Frequency of inventory counts and dates are set by the CFO. Drug pricing is determined by the DoP, but approved by the CFO.

Pharmaceutical pricing for patient charging is a dynamic process that requires hyper-vigilance by the DoP. Charges for pharmaceuticals are maintained in databases referred to as the charge data master (CDM) or charge master. Inventory costs are constantly changing and will require related charges be updated frequently. The goal is to keep a profit margin that is above the cost of goods and to meet a predefined profit margin. The profit margin is defined as the difference between sale price and purchase price. Determining drug mark-up formulas requires an analysis of desired net revenue from the sell of goods. Net revenue is defined as the cost of goods minus expenses incurred to purchase, stock, and dispense merchandise.

There is not one set way to determine sale price of goods in the pharmacy. A couple of ways to calculate the sale price are using the Average Wholesale Price (AWP) times a multiplier for all goods or by multiplying the AWP by different multipliers for each type of supply or medication.

More complicated markup formulas will have different multipliers per supply type and purchase price ranges. Market averages and/or calculated overhead expenses per supply stat determine multipliers.

An example of a markup formula may be as follows:

Oral Drugs	Injectables	Compounds	Non-drug supplies
3 x AWP	4 x AWP	2 x AWP of all components + dispensing fee	2 x acquisition cost

Accounting

Departments of the hospital are classified by Accounting in one of two ways, as Cost Centers (CC) or Revenue Centers (RC). Cost Centers are departments that generate expenses, but do not produce revenue. Examples of CCs are Environmental Services or Facilities Management Departments, which are internal departments that maintain hospital functions without creating a revenue stream. Revenue Centers have operation expenses, but also produce revenue. An example of a RC would be the Surgery Department, which has operational expenses and surgical patient revenue.

Inpatient Pharmacies can be defined either as a CC or RC depending on the services provided and designation of the CFO. The Pharmacy Department could be deemed a CC if medications are considered an expense that is deducted from lump sum payment for a given diagnosis. If the Pharmacy provides other non-dispensing services that are billable, such as ambulatory services, then the Pharmacy Department can be designated as a RC.

Knowing the Pharmacy's designation as a CC or RC can help determine how to manage inventories, develop new services and how to communicate this information to the CFO. If the pharmacy is a CC, it will be even more important to control cost of goods. A designation of RC will not eliminate the need to control cost of goods, but will allow for new services to create additional revenue sources. A designation of RC is more desirable in terms of effectiveness for the DoP to gain budget approval for any new pharmacy services.

DoPs can affect Accounts Payable (AP) much more than Accounts Receivable (AR) due to the fact that AR is dependent on hospital volumes while AP is based on expenses. AP are expenses owed to outside vendors that the hospital must pay within a defined time frame to receive best pricing, discounts and to avoid late charges and/or penalties. Daily vigilance in receiving drugs, supplies and other goods is essential to maintaining AP. Expense control is a major role of a DoP.

AR are charges to vendors and patients that are potential revenue for the hospital. DoPs are responsible for the proper billing, maintenance of drug and service charges, but actual collection is usually a duty of the Accounting Department. Other considerations would be proper coding of medications to assist in proper insurance billing, further discussion of coding will be found in the informatics chapter. The pharmacy has minimal effect on hospital volumes depending on services provided.

Sarbanes-Oxley (SOX) anti-fraud regulations are accounting rules that do not allow a single individual to order, receive and pay for products. These rules must be followed to avoid prosecution and/or fines. The CFO will monitor compliance to SOX regulations.

Inventory is the accounting of all drugs and supplies on hand. A physical count of the inventory is usually scheduled annually, but can be more frequent at the discretion of the CFO. The annual inventory is the time of year that the DoP can show how well they are managing supply costs. Good inventory control is achieved through daily vigilance and not by casual observance. Having a dedicated Buyer position will streamline inventory and ensure over/under-stocking is minimized. Contract compliance is also essential to controlling cost of goods. A good Buyer can quickly pay for their position by adhering to contract purchasing. Annual inventory can be performed by the pharmacy staff or by an outside contracted vendor, depending on staffing needs and cost considerations. Automation is very helpful in maintaining perpetual inventories, but often times are luxuries not readily available in many smaller hospitals.

Revenue reports are generated daily by the Accounting and Pharmacy information systems. It is best practice to reconcile these reports daily to make sure all charges were found in both systems. By reconciling these reports daily the DoP can become familiar with drug charges, coding, missed charges, charging errors and volumes. Reviewing charges is also a SOX requirement and the reconciled reports are required to be on hand for a designated period of time. The CFO may require the reconciled reports be sent to them for review and filing.

Each month every hospital department should receive a Departmental Operations Report (DOR). This report shows all gross revenue and expenses. The revenue is based on volumes which the DoP has little or no control over. The only change the DoP can make on revenue is at the pricing level of drugs and services. Expenses are affected by the DoP's monthly constant vigilance of inventory control, contract adherence, and human resource management. DORs compare budgeted revenue and expenses to actual charges and expenses. All expenses should be reviewed for accuracy and any disputed charges reported to Accounting for review. It is the duty of the DoP to provide action plans to correct numbers over/under budget to the Controller monthly.

Chapter 2

Productivity

Other information available in the DOR is productivity and human resource management information. For example, the total number of hours worked or full-time equivalents (FTE) budgeted versus actual is reported. Again, variance reports will require explanations and action plans to be developed for correction. The DoP's direct supervisor and CFO closely scrutinize these reports. The DoP manages staffing to ensure coverage stays within the defined budget parameters.

DORs also show the number of medications dispensed, which is defined as a stat for reporting. Stats are a measure of inventory velocity and inventory turnover to determine productivity. Inventory turns refers to the calculation of an estimated number of times the whole pharmacy's inventory is sold and replaced within a given time period. Inventory turns are used as a measure to determine the efficiency of inventory management. The goal is to turn the inventory more and more frequently. By measuring the stat volumes the CFO can determine the number of FTEs the pharmacy will need to manage the calculated volumes. Another tool the CFO uses to determine staffing needs is the man-hours per stat (man-hours/stat) calculation. The man-hours/stat results, attempt to standardize the total stat volume, which can be compared to other hospital pharmacies of similar size within the enterprise (if applicable) to determine efficiencies. DoPs need to ensure they understand how the stat is defined at their facility and how it is used. By knowing how the stat is defined the DoP can make sure all drugs in the computerized formulary database are set up correctly. If formulary items are not properly built in the database then drugs that should be dispensed as multiple stats per dispensing, could mistakenly be recorded as one stat per dispensing, thereby report lower productivity numbers than desired. Decisions made on faulty stats may lead to below par staffing, and employee dissatisfaction. Incorrect stats will create final billing errors that could result in unintended fraudulent billing to CMS and other insurance carriers, which may lead to refunds and possible fines.

Some facilities may have software that measures daily FTEs used to assist managers in maintaining staffing at or below budget. If the DoP has access to productivity software, then it is incumbent upon he/she to monitor this information daily and make any necessary adjustments in staffing to remain within the allocated FTEs. Where no productivity software exists, routine processes should be developed to monitor productivity daily.

Knowing accounting terminology will be essential for the DoP to review financial reports. General Ledger (GL) reports show all revenue and expense line items. Each main GL account may have multiple detailed accounts, which are referred to as subGL accounts. General ledgers are divided into Revenue and Expense sections that will have columns for budgeted and actual values. Revenue will show all revenue sources and total gross revenue. Gross revenue is the sum of all revenue sources before expenses. It is important to note that gross revenue reflects billed income not received income. Net revenue is income minus expenses and appears on the GL as the last line or better known as "the bottom line". It is the net revenue that will determine profit or loss for the given time period. Each month's financial outcomes are reported as month-to-date (MTD) and the yearly sum each month is referred to as the year-to-date (YTD) totals. These totals should be used to compare to the previous years outcomes to determine current financial progress.

Expenses are also delineated on the GL, and are more directly impacted by the DoP, than is revenue. The DoP should monitor all expenses monthly to determine his/her effectiveness in managing day-to-day operation expenses. As inventory and FTE's are managed, it will be evident where changes need to be made to improve adherence to the budgeted goals.

Chapter 3

Budget

Pharmacy capital and operational budgeting is the responsibility of the DoP. When discussing the budget, DoPs must know the difference between fiscal and calendar year. The fiscal year can be the same as the calendar year, but often times the fiscal year does not start in January. The fiscal year is the twelve months for which the capital and operational budgets are calculated, set and monitored. Each fiscal year the DoP will be asked to submit operational and capital equipment budget requests.

Operational budgets are estimates of all departmental expenses that will be incurred for daily operations for the next fiscal year. Operational expenses include salaries, benefits, drug inventory costs, drug supplies, office supplies, utilities, shipping costs, etc. Monitoring of these expenses are reported on the DOR and variance reports. Variance reports are accounting reports that are provided to departmental directors for review and explanation. These reports show the actual revenue and expenses compared to the budgeted revenue and expenses. Overages and shortages must be explained on the variance report and submitted to the CFO or their designee. By submitting a completed Variance Report to the CFO, the DoP keeps an open line of communication between the Pharmacy and the CFO, which allows the DoP to clearly communicate successes and needs.

The budget becomes a working document for the DoP to guide management of expenses month-to-month. Actual expenses should be less than budgeted expenses; budgets should not be viewed as a spending goal. Annual Operational Budgets will be developed from the previous years actual expenses plus any growth estimates and new service cost projections.

Capital Budgets are performed annually and are used for capital equipment costs. Like the Operational Budgets, the Capital Budget is created each fiscal year. Unlike the Operational Budget the Capital Budget is not used as a month-to-month working document. The Capital Budget requires the DoP to submit his/her capital equipment requests once annually with a clear explanation of the equipment need. It is recommended that all explanations include a Return on Investment (ROI) or break-even analysis, when appropriate, to improve the possibility of approval. Once the CFO receives all the departmental capital requests, equipment purchases are prioritized based on the facility's overall allocated Capital Equipment Budget?

Chapter 4

Human Resources

Human Resources (HR) refers to the department's employees and their needs. A whole department exists for the management of HR. It is beyond the scope of this training to discuss all aspects of HR management. A DoP must make his/herself well versed in HR management as they are in a management role requiring supervision of employees. Good understanding of HR regulations or knowledge of where and when to ask for assistance from an HR expert is essential. Without this understanding the DoP can put the facility and themselves at a legal risk. It is recommended that the DoP consult their HR department for information on hiring, disciplining, leave, or terminating employees. Other areas that will require an HR consult are in regard to leaves of absence that require completion of Family Medical Leave Act (FMLA) paperwork.

Human Resources expenses are the number one expense of the Pharmacy Department, thereby requiring hyper-vigilance by the DoP. Hiring the proper people and keeping the best employees should be the goal of management. High turnover of employees increases cost and depletes talent and operational knowledge, which leads to insufficient department operations and lowers employee morale.

Only high performing employees should remain on staff to provide safe care for the patients, maintain high performance, ensure adherence to regulations and for overall ease of HR management. High performers are employees that do not need constant direction, who are self motivated, proactive, creative, manageable, conscientious, honest, pleasant and who have an impeccable work ethic. The DoP can delegate duties and assignments to high performers with confidence that the tasks will be completed in a timely manner.

Employees that are not high performers will not be tolerated by high performers and will require intervention by the DoP. Lack of action by management to correct subpar employees will be seen by others, as acceptance of poor behavior and performance. A permissive environment that allows for low performance is not an environment high performers will tolerate. Unacceptable behavior that is permitted we be perceived as acceptable and will perpetuate future poor behavior.

The Pharmacy Department has some of the most highly educated and trained employees in the hospital. Due to the nature of the work of hospital pharmacy employees, the DoP must develop methods to train and record training of his/her employees to meet regulatory standards, keep knowledge base up-to-date and to improve employee satisfaction. Training can develop employees into high performers, if the employee has the desire to improve. Substandard employees should be improved to achieve high performance and increase productivity, or dismissed.

Employee development and job satisfaction are key roles of the DoP. Longevity of employees, if managed appropriately, will decrease costs and increase productivity and efficiency. Recruiting and training is not only difficult it is expensive in regards to monetary costs and knowledge loss. As mentioned, employee development is one tool for employee satisfaction, but there are several tools that can be used to increase employee satisfaction. Reward and recognition both formal and informal are great ways to improve morale. Employees that are appreciated tend to work harder and support management.

Flexible scheduling and a deliberate effort to award time off when requested is key to employee satisfaction. A DoP should approach managing people as if they serve the employee and not the other way around. DoPs that are willing to step up and do the daily work activities performed by his or her staff gain much more respect then do those that are not willing to help.

Communication is the biggest factor in management and employee relations. Lack of communication, at all levels will lead to job dissatisfaction and to a possible credibility gap between management and staff. Always be honest and upfront with employees even when sharing disappointing or undesirable information. Be kind and never be personal when having to reprimand or redirect employees no matter how hard the discussion becomes or if the employee makes the discussion personal. Keep employees informed of their performance expectations frequently and not just at annual reviews.

DoPs who work closely with their staff should develop a keen understanding of their employees' skills, likes, dislikes and areas of expertise. By understanding the individual employee's skill sets, the DoP can assign duties to those individuals that can best achieve their assignment and allow them to derive job satisfaction from their accomplishments. Employees that find satisfaction in their work are naturally more productive.

Pharmacy Informatics includes electronic recording of healthcare information, development of electronic clinical decision support material, and the maintenance of all computerized systems related to the ordering, stocking, dispensing, charging and administering of medications. The DoP's role in Pharmacy Informatics depends on staffing and/or the DoP's computer skill set. Larger departments may have an Informatics Pharmacist who the DoP will oversee, but more commonly the DoP will be directly involved in monitoring, building, and maintaining Pharmacy Information Systems (PIS).

The main role of the DoP is to maintain the integrity of the PIS databases. Pharmacy Information Systems have several databases which include the formulary, frequency tables, drug route tables, reason tables, charge master files and unit of measure tables to name a few. Many of these databases do not require extensive time requirements to maintain once initially built. The formulary database requires constant vigilance due to the dynamic nature of a formulary system. Delegation by the DoP to a competent pharmacy employee can be done, as long as the DoP maintains his/her knowledge of the process and monitors changes.

Medication management Clinical Decision Support (CDS) settings in the Electronic Health Record (EHR) software must be reviewed by the DoP and discussed with medical staff in the appropriate committees. CDS rules will determine the level of alerts that will be viewed by the providers during order entry and will affect provider adoption of Computerized Provider Order Entry (CPOE), if implemented at the facility. DoPs or their designee should be well versed in Meaningful Use (MU) requirements if there facility is participating in the US Government's HITECH Act reimbursement program.

It is important to note that maintaining the CDM database will require a thorough understanding of billing, coding, and insurance regulations. Understanding the payer mix and what the different payers reimburse helps the DoP evaluate if current pharmacy services or new potential services are feasible.

Automation is another area of informatics. Like the PIS it is very important that the DoP have an extensive understanding of the functionality and setup of the Automated Dispensing Cabinets (ADC). Understanding functionally of the ADC will allow the DoP to develop efficient workflows, policies, security models, and reports necessary to monitor use and fulfill regulations. Again, the formulary maintenance of the ADC can be delegated, and is recommended, as long as the DoP keeps his/her skills up-to-date and frequently reviews changes to ensure updates are being made. Part of the DoP oversight should be monitoring policy and workflow adherence by pharmacy staff. It is important to communicate the policies and develop workflow monitoring tools for staff to encourage compliance to written policies and workflow designs. Due to the physical capacity of the ADC the inventory becomes a budget concern; therefore the DoP should be involved in the setting of par levels and what drugs are stocked. Periodic ADC inventories and usage audits by the DoP or designee should be performed to maintain inventory control.

Smart pump drug libraries are another area of informatics that is under the DoP's purview. Proper intravenous pump drug setup is essential in the safe and proper use of the smart pump. Although the maintenance of the pump drug library is not as involved as other drug libraries once built, it is as crucial to monitor the pump use to determine possible additions, deletions or changes to the pump drug library. Errors in the drug library can cause harm to a patient because the pump is used for drug administration not drug dispensing. Due to these safety concerns, delegation of the drug library is discouraged and collaboration with another clinical pharmacist is encouraged.

Bar code scanning as it relates to medication management is another informatics duty of the DoP. The success of bedside Bar Code Medication Administration (BCMA) is incumbent upon the medication's bar code scanning. Processes for ensuring that medications' bar codes scan, should be developed. For example, bar code scanning all drugs received from vendors in the pharmacy can help to find drugs that do not scan prior to distribution. Reporting methodologies and routines should be set in place for the end user to report any scanning failures to allow for a prompt resolution.

Education on new software and updates to existing software is another role of the DoP or designee. Well planned training materials and communication of training to all pertinent staff is essential to the successful roll out of new software or updates.

The DoP should be involved with any committees that will be considering software changes that will affect medication management within the facility to ensure all regulations, standards, policies and procedures, and proper medication use practices are met prior to implementation.

Chapter 6

Regulation

There are several regulating bodies that the DoP must be aware of and well versed in their roles as they pertain to pharmacy operations. The main regulators are Centers for Medicare and Medicaid Services (CMS), Office of Inspector General (OIG), Accreditation Organization, State Board of Pharmacy and DEA. The CMS is the Federal Government Department that sets conditions of participation (CoP) by which the hospital must meet to receive payment from the Federal Government insurance programs. It is important to note that a large percentage of revenue for many hospitals is provide by the government programs and maintaining the ability to participate in the programs is mandatory for the success of these hospitals. The OIG is the enforcement arm of CMS and will provide the inspectors for evaluation of compliance to the conditions.

Hospitals voluntarily contract with accreditation organizations that are recognized by CMS as compliance review agents for Condition of Participation (CoP) in Medicare and Medicaid programs. Reviewing CMS CoP is not the only reason for these Accreditation Organizations. These organizations provide quality standards by which the hospitals must comply to be accredited. Accreditation is recognized by insurance providers and is a symbol of quality that can be displayed and advertised. Failure to become accredited puts the hospital at risk for substantial revenue loss and credibility damage, so the emphasis on accreditation cannot be over stated. The Joint Commission (JC) is the most commonly contracted accreditation organization, but there are others that are recognized by CMS. DoPs should be highly versed in the hospital's accreditation organization's medication management standards. Pharmacy Directors should be able to provide required documentation when requested by accreditation surveyors and be able to speak to current policies and procedures as they pertain to accreditation standards.

Most DoPs understand the Board of Pharmacy (BoP) is their state regulatory body and must be an expert on state pharmacy law. A BoP inspector can arrive at the pharmacy any time to enforce state pharmacy regulation. It is recommended that the DoP maintain pharmacy operations at regulatory and accreditation standards at all times and not live in fear of possible inspections. DoPs are usually the Pharmacist-in-Charge (PIC) and responsible for all state and federal pharmacy law adherence, but can delegate this designation to a trusted staff Registered Pharmacist as regulations allow.

Drug security, diversion avoidance and recording are the responsibility of the PIC. The Federal Drug Administration (FDA) and the Drug Enforcement Agency (DEA) set and enforce regulation for medications, including controlled substances. Prescription drug and controlled substance ordering, storing, recording and dispensing regulations are also set by and enforced by the DEA. The DoP must know the Federal regulations and ensure compliance at all times, even if the DoP is not the PIC who is legally responsible. By being well versed in regulation compliance and knowing the current adherence status the DoP will be prepared to answer questions concerning regulatory issues from their direct supervisor and to participate intelligently in investigations that may arise. Being prepared to discuss regulatory status will relieve the DoP of concerns of legal issues that will arise.

Chapter 7

Quality

Quality measures span the topics of regulation, finance, patient care, accreditation, and continuous improvement. Hospitals have developed a whole department for quality control and the Quality Director is responsible for maintaining quality standards set by government regulatory departments and accreditation organizations. DoPs should develop several key performance indicators (KPI) for the Pharmacy Department. A KPI should be measurable and useful to the improvement of a process or function of the pharmacy. Quality dashboards may be developed to assist the DoP in organizing clinical, financial, regulatory, and operation quality measures. Dashboards are very useful for recording and reporting quality measures. Each quality measure should be trended to determine any need for change. When a change in current processes is determined by the KPI an action plan should be developed to correct the finding as part of the continuous improvement process. Each hospital will adopt a continuous improvement model, of which there are several. For example the Plan Do Study Act (PDSA) model is commonly used. This model refers to the process of quality improvement. "Plan" in this model is the development of an action plan as previously mentioned. "Do" is the implementation of the plan. "Study" refers to the review of outcomes and "Act" is the implementation of positive outcomes as a new and improved process. Documentation of these quality processes is essential to communicate actions to senior management, governing bodies and accreditation surveyors.

Chapter 8

Medication Management

Medication management as discussed in this chapter refers to the procurement, stocking, recording, storing, expiring, wasting and dispensing medication. Procurement of medications and assurance of drug supply is one of the DoP's primary roles. Due to the importance of this duty the DoP must be very well versed in ordering processes.

The majority of ordering is performed via the primary wholesaler. Ordering via the primary wholesaler will maintain drug pedigrees and proper contract pricing. Although the wholesaler has some contracts or discount pricing the majority is negotiated and maintained by the General Purchasing Organization (GPO). Once the contracts are negotiated and executed the information is supplied to the wholesaler for implementation. Each year the GPO will review the contract pricing and renegotiate prices, which is called a "bid role". When these prices are updated the DoP must make sure the prices are updates in the CDM to make sure charges reflect updated cost and desired margins.

When medications are not available, other ordering avenues need to be in place. Some of these avenues are asking the wholesaler to check other distribution center, ordering from a secondary contracted wholesaler (if available), direct ordering from the manufacturer, local pharmacy relationships and secondary market vendors.

Wholesalers are organized into regional distribution centers (DC) whose primary customers are within their defined region. Due to this priority it is often difficult convince the wholesaler to search DCs outside the designated DC, but this still remains as a first option to secure a allocated or back ordered medication. When contracted medications are not supplied by the primary wholesaler it is important to check to see if their is a failure to supply clause in the contract. If a failure to supply clause exists then the wholesaler is required to reimburse the pharmacy for the cost difference for acquiring the drug from a secondary source or a non-contract substitution.

Rarely, hospitals will have primary and secondary drug wholesalers. If a secondary wholesaler is available then they become a viable option to procure back ordered medication. Usually the secondary wholesaler's pricing will not be at the primary wholesaler's contract pricing, but the drug origin integrity is known.

Invoice management is another essential duty of the DoP. Knowing the pay cycle will allow for timely payments of invoices and avoids late charges. Terms of payment often state a certain percent discount when invoice totals are paid within a designated time frame. Good invoice management will ensure best purchase pricing.

Direct from the manufacturer purchasing is common when the product in question is allocated by the manufacturer. Buying direct requires the hospital to have an account with the manufacturer. The Materials Management Director would be a good contact to determine if a business relationship exists or to start the process of developing one.

Drug shortages or ordering errors are an everyday event in hospital pharmacy practice. Planning for these events requires good relationships with other local hospitals and pharmacies. Having trading partners allows for same day procurement when necessary.

Another way to ensure drug supply is asking the patient to supply their own drug for those rarely used home non-formulary medications that are ordered to continue upon admission. This situation must be handled by the proper procedure as defined by policy.

Inventory management requires the DoP to set goals for par and max levels. Automated dispensing cabinet inventory levels should also be at the direction of the DoP. Once inventory level guidelines are set the DoP can assign their Buyer to maintain inventory as defined. Although the inventory maintenance is assigned to the buyer, the DoP should have accountability measures in place to ensure proper adherence to inventory goals.

Maintaining the integrity of the current inventory of medications is another responsibility of the DoP/PIC. Policies and procedures should be developed to monitor for expired, degraded, or improperly stored medications. Proper security of the medications inside and outside the pharmacy is under the purview of the PIC. The policies should be detailed and provide clear instructions on how and when drug inventories are inspected, how drugs are stored, expired or recalled. Logs should be developed to record storage temperatures where appropriate and to record drug recall actions. Although pharmacy technicians are responsible for the day-to-day activities, accountability and reporting measures must be in place to communicate progress and completion to the PIC. Undocumented inspections should be deemed as not performed and will not satisfy regulation. Without proper documentation the PIC cannot provide necessary evidence to regulatory or accreditation surveyors. The PIC must review all documentation and communicate their review to staff to make sure the importance of the documentation is well understood. By emphasizing the review of the documentation it ensures better adherence to policy and procedure.

Expired medications shall be removed from inventory and stored in a clearly marked area to avoid dispensing of expired medications. All state and federal regulations regarding expired medication return and destruction should be followed when disposing of expired or degraded medications.

Medication recalls are frequent and require processes and proper documentations. Recall logs must contain the level of recall and actions taken and will stand as a record for regulation and a historic record.

Chapter 9

Clinical Duties

Clinical responsibilities often times fall to the DoP, when a Clinical Manager is not feasible. Clinical programs are an area where the pharmacy can show cost savings. Developing new clinical programs and Pharmacy & Therapeutics Committee agendas are other clinical duties of the DoP.

Some of the clinical programs that can be developed are therapeutic interchange, IV/PO switch, pharmacokinetic dosing, anti-microbial stewardship, renal dosing and anti-coagulation. In-services for pharmacy staff, medical staff and nursing staff are more opportunities for clinical programs. Focusing on CMS Core Measures and joining ASHP to keep current with pharmacists' changing roles in Pharmacy Practice will assist in developing new clinical practice programs.

Often hospital pharmacies will have pharmacy school students, which require the DoP or designee to be a preceptor at a local Pharmacy School. If it is decided that the hospital pharmacy will accept students for clinical rotations, then time should be allocated to instruct the students, train the preceptor and a syllabus should be developed to clearly define what is expected of the student. Having students helps the pharmacists stay current with their clinical knowledge and provides a recruitment tool through networking with the students and local Pharmacy Schools. Make sure all HR requirements are met prior to signing students up for rotations.

Chapter 10

New Positions and Programs

As Pharmacy operations are developed and change over time new programs and new positions will need to be developed. There are several considerations that need to be addressed when creating new positions or programs. First, the needs of a new position or program should be clearly defined and listed. Once the need is defined, a list of implementation steps must be delineated and become a part of a business proposal. In the business proposal there must be precise explanation of the need for the new position or program, backed by statistical facts and proposed benefits to the organization. A Return on Investment (ROI) should be calculated and be a part of any proposal where appropriate.

ROI calculations are evaluations of costs to develop, implement, and maintain a new position or program, and an estimate of the time needed to regain all costs incurred for the implementation of the new position. For example, if a new position for a Pharmacy Buyer was going to be proposed the ROI may be calculated as follows:

Expenses (all calculations are for illustration purposes only)

Wages - $16 per hour x 2080 = $33,280

Benefits - (0.25 x $33,280) = $8,320 (Check with HR for benefit costs)

Total = $41,600 annual expenses

Revenue

Current inventory cost $200,000

Current Annual Drug Spend $500,000

Current contract compliance 75%

Estimate contract compliance w/Buyer 80%, 90%, 100%

Current lost savings from contract non-compliance (real data comes from GPO reports, but for this example % non-compliance x current drug spend was used). $500,000 x 0.25 = $125,000 annually.

Potential Improved Contract Compliance Savings

Contract Compliance	80%	90%	100%
Savings	$25,000	$75,000	$125,000

Estimated inventory reduction goal 25% or $50,000 over 5 years.

Potential five-year savings range

Inventory Savings/ Contract Savings %	Year 1	Year 2	Year 3	Year 4	Year 5	Total Savings
80%	$30,000	$30,000	$30,000	$30,000	$30,000	$150,000
90%	$80,000	$80,000	$80,000	$80,000	$80,000	$400,000
100%	$130,000	$130,000	$130,000	$130,000	$130,000	$650,000

Note: Each year would be less and less savings as the new baseline inventory is approach. Above example shows simple percentages for illustration only.

By taking the total revenue potential per year and dividing by the total expenses per year to implement the position or program will determine the ROI. For the example above, if the lowest savings were to be used to be conservative the calculation would be ($41,600/$30,000) x 1 year = 1.38 years ~ 1.4 years or 1.4 years x 12 months/year = 16.8 month for an ROI. In other words, it will take 16.8 month for the hospital to regain the total cost of their investment to implement a Pharmacy Buyer position.

Chapter 11

Daily Operations

The importance of the involvement of the DoP in developing the guidelines for daily pharmacy operations is essential to efficient pharmacy operations. Development of clear and concise departmental policies and procedures will increase adherence to defined workflows and procedures to achieve desired outcomes. Allowing the pharmacy staff to develop their own workflows and daily processes is not recommended and is hard to correct, if necessary, once implemented. Constant evaluation of new procedures is required to ensure the staff is compliant to the procedure. Without supervision and accountability old habits will return and new processes will fail. Development of written or electronic logs to record daily performance is good visual tools to determine adherence to proper procedures.

Large facilities may benefit from a Pharmacy Operations Manager to assist with daily operations like scheduling, staffing, payroll and daily duties management. Operational duties for smaller facilities are the responsibility of the DoP.

One of the DoP's most time consuming duties is attending meetings. The Pharmacy is responsible for the content of the Pharmacy and Therapeutic Committee (P&T) and co-chairs the committee. Other committees that may require pharmacy involvement are Accreditation, Quality, Leadership, Safety, Infection Control, ICU to name a few. Due to the number of committee meetings the DoP can appoint staff pharmacists to committees. By assigning staff to committees for which the individual has expertise the DoP can better manage human resources and their own time. Utilizing pharmacist for committee involvement and clinical duties can lead to better job satisfaction for the high performing employee.

Chapter 12

Communication

Due to the leadership role the DoP holds they must have excellent written and oral communication skills. Communicating with Physicians and executives can be very intimidating and frequently very frustrating. When communicating with physicians and/or executives one must always be respectful and approach the conversation from the physician's and/or executive's point of view. There will be times when the DoP will have to be firm and non-compromising due to regulations, patient safety, or personal ethics, but being willing to listen and work towards a win-win solution for the benefit of all involved is a very good skill to develop. When conversations become combative or personal it is time to end the conversation as professionally as possible to regroup and develop a new approach.

It is important to remember the DoP is responsible for medication management and is the gatekeeper of medication use and procurement for the hospital. Good communication of the formulary, shortages, recalls and substitutions is key to a compliant medical staff. If the culture around the medical staff and Pharmacy Department is adversarial, accomplishing pharmacy initiatives will be very difficult. The DoP must remember the physicians are the revenue source for the hospital, while balancing their role as medication manager. When the medical staff trusts the knowledge of the pharmacists and values their input, pharmacist involvement in patient care increases.

Nursing and pharmacy relations should also be one of cooperation and understanding. Often times hospitals struggle with the nursing and pharmacy relationships. Pharmacists and nurses do not speak the same language often times and struggle to understand each other's points of view. Due to the shear number of nurses compared to pharmacists in a hospital and the fact the CNO may oversee Nursing and Pharmacy Departments the DoP must work well with Nursing or the will not be effective managers. Developing working relationships with Nursing leaders is essential to the success of a DoP.

Glossary of Terms

340B Program - Federal Government program that allows qualified pharmacies to purchase medications at a reduced cost for outpatient dispensing in disproportionate share designated communities.

ADC - Average Daily Census or Automated Dispensing Cabinet

APD - Adjusted Patient Days

BCMA - Bar Code Medication Administration

Capital Budget - a written estimate of future expenses that will incur due to purchase or maintenance of new or existing equipment or tangible resources.

CDM - Charge Data Master File (charge master)

CDS - Clinical Decision Support

CMS - Centers for Medicare and Medicaid

COB - Close of Business

CoP - Conditions of Participation

CPOE - Computerized Provider Order Entry/Computerized Physician Order Entry

Daily Revenue (End-of-Day) Report - a daily revenue report generated by the department information system that indicates items dispensed for the given day and the respective revenue charged.

DoP- Director of Pharmacy

DOR- Department Operations Report

EHR - Electronic Health Record

EOD - End of Day

FMLA - Family Medical Leave Act

FTE - Full-Time Equivalent

GL - General Ledger

GPO - General Purchasing Organization

Gross Revenue - all billed revenue prior to deducting expenses and taxes.

KPI - Key Performance Indicator

IDN - integrated delivery network

LOS - Length of Stay

MHS - Man-hours per Stat

MU - Meaningful Use requirement set by CMS that must be met to participate in the US Government's HITECH Act reimbursement program.

Net Revenue - all revenue after deducting expenses and taxes

Operational Budget - a written estimate of future expenses that will be incurred due to daily business operations.

PI - Performance Improvement

PIS - Pharmacy Information System

P&T Committee - Pharmacy and Therapeutics Committee

Revenue/Stat Report - a daily accounting report, which indicates the number of stats dispensed, and the associated charges that crossed to the Accounting software from the Pharmacy software.

ROI -Return on Investment (Break Even Analysis)

Secondary Supplies - pharmaceutical supplier that secondary to the primary wholesaler and is used as a backup supply source.

SOX -Sarbanes/Oxley Accounting Regulations

Stat - a defined measure of productivity (i.e. Number of doses dispensed)

Sub GL - individual account subcategories within the general ledger

Variance Report - an accounting report that is required to explain differences between budgeted expectations and actual outcomes.

Wholesaler - medication supplier that adheres to the GPO contracts, and is the main source of pharmaceutical and supplies.